Betsey MacDonald
~ 92 ~

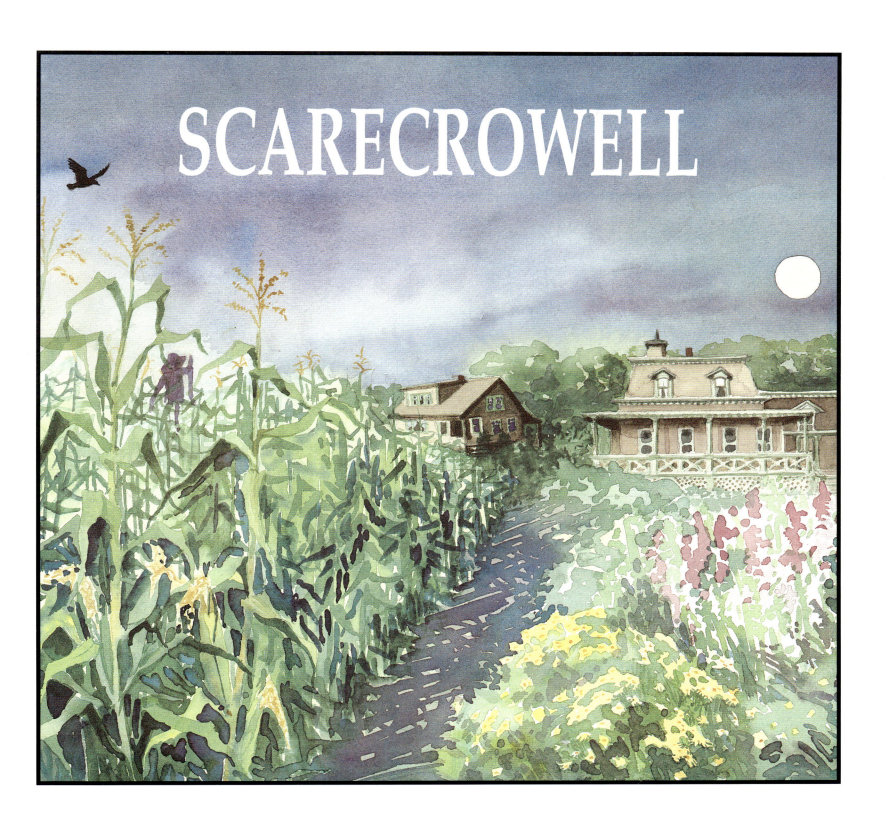

SCARECROWELL

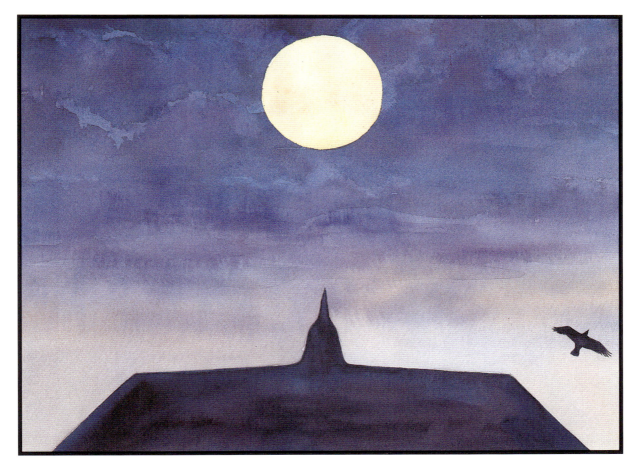

BETSEY DOUGLAS MACDONALD

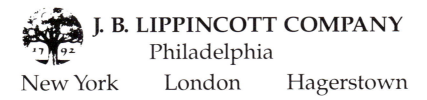

J. B. LIPPINCOTT COMPANY
Philadelphia
New York   London   Hagerstown

For My Mom

6 5 4 3 2 1

Library of Congress Cataloging-in-Publication Data

MacDonald, Betsey Douglas.
    Scarecrowell : story and paintings / by Betsey Douglas MacDonald.
      p.   cm.
    Summary: Nathaniel is afraid of his neighbor, old Mrs. Crowell, until she befriends him and shares the beauty of her garden with him.
    ISBN 0-397-51261-9
    [1. Old age—Fiction.   2. Fear—Fiction.   3. Gardening—Fiction.]
I. Title.
PZ7.M14637Sc   1992
[E]—dc20

91–30001
CIP
AC

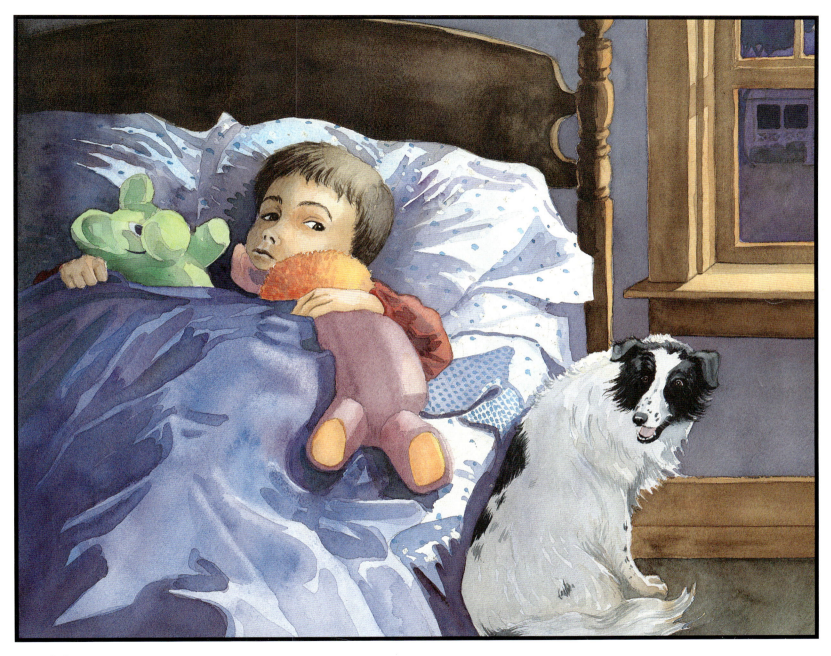

Nathaniel's eyes were wide open. He couldn't sleep because the moon was too bright and shadows were moving around his room. He knew the shadows were from old Mrs. Crowell's trees, but that made them even creepier.

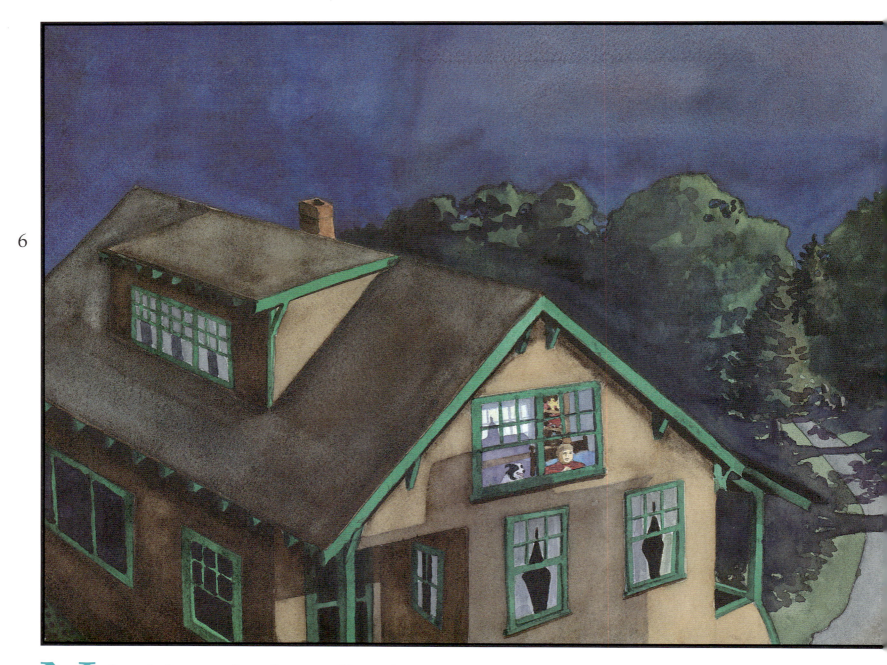

Nathaniel stared at his wall and, as he did, one shadow began to grow. It pointed towards the ceiling. Then it spread out and began to look like an enormous ebony crow.

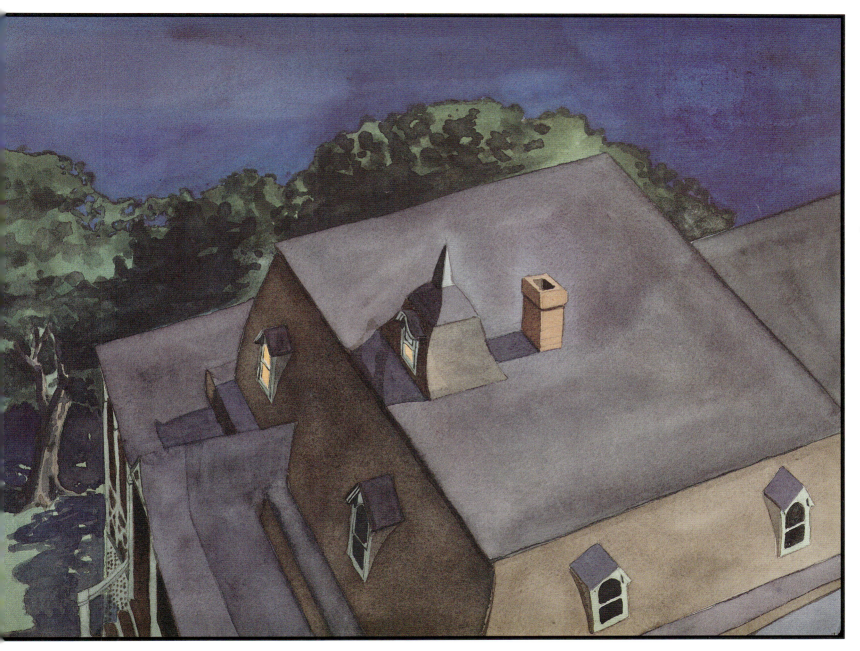

Even though he was frightened, Nathaniel crept to his window and peeked over the sill. But all he could see was the roof of old Mrs. Crowell's house. Then a cloud erased the moon's light, and the crow shadow disappeared. Nathaniel went back to bed and fell asleep.

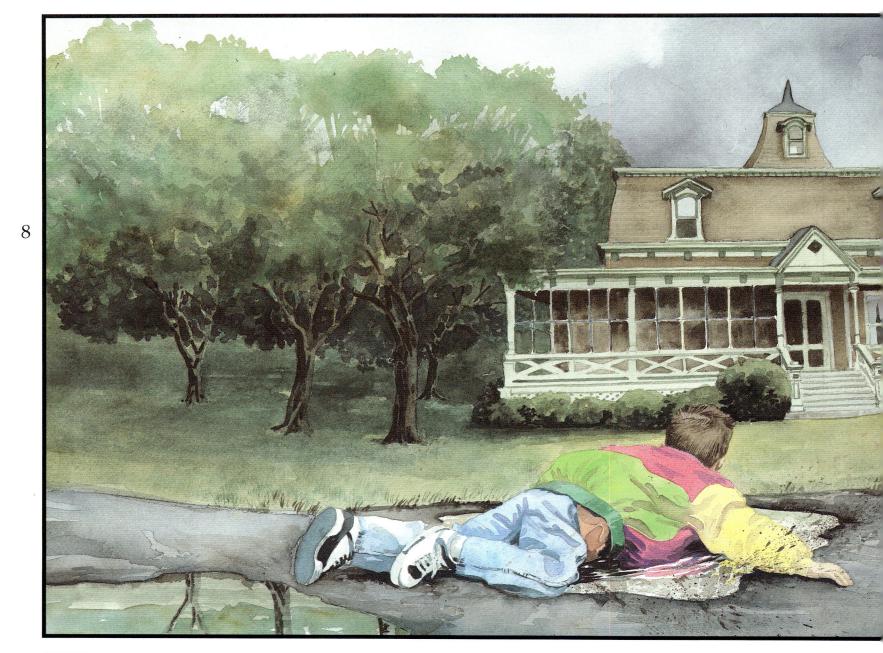

The morning was gray and drizzly, but Nathaniel's dog, Jeff, needed to go for a walk. Nathaniel put on his favorite pink, yellow, green, and purple windbreaker, the old one that his mother wanted to throw away. He didn't look at old Mrs. Crowell's house as he walked by, but he thought he saw something black moving in the yard.

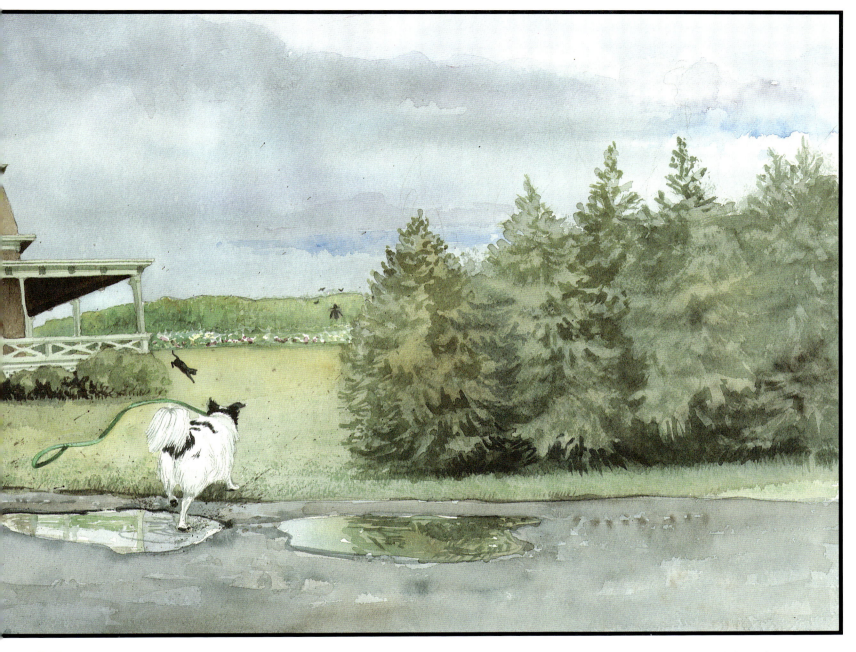

Jeff saw it, too. He went wild! It was old Mrs. Crowell's black cat, Shadow. Shadow ran across the porch, over the railing, and into the backyard. Jeff ran after her. Nathaniel slipped and fell in some mud.

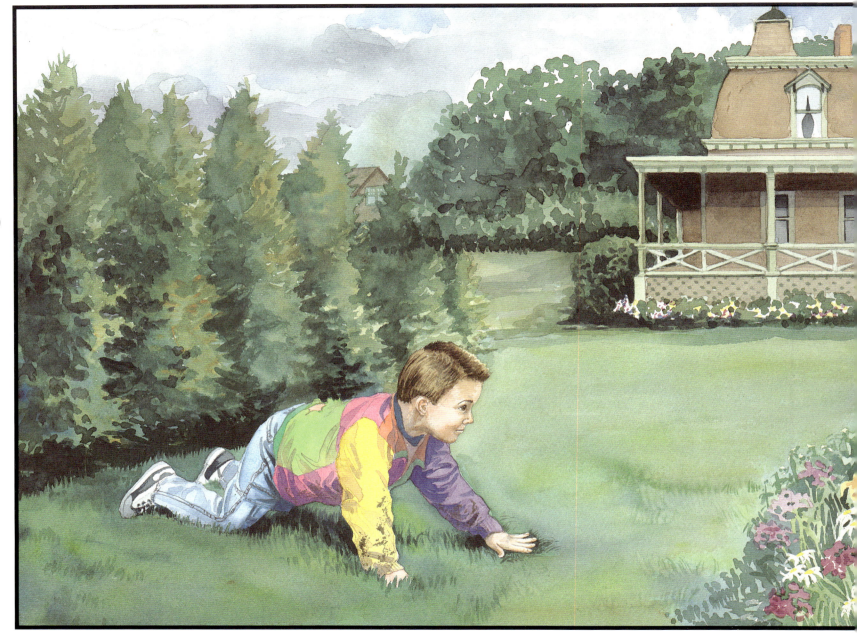

e didn't know why, but Nathaniel was afraid of old Mrs. Crowell. So he crawled through the hedge and crept into her backyard. What a backyard it was! There were plants, flowers, and gardens everywhere. Jeff and Shadow were drinking from a birdbath in the middle of the yard.

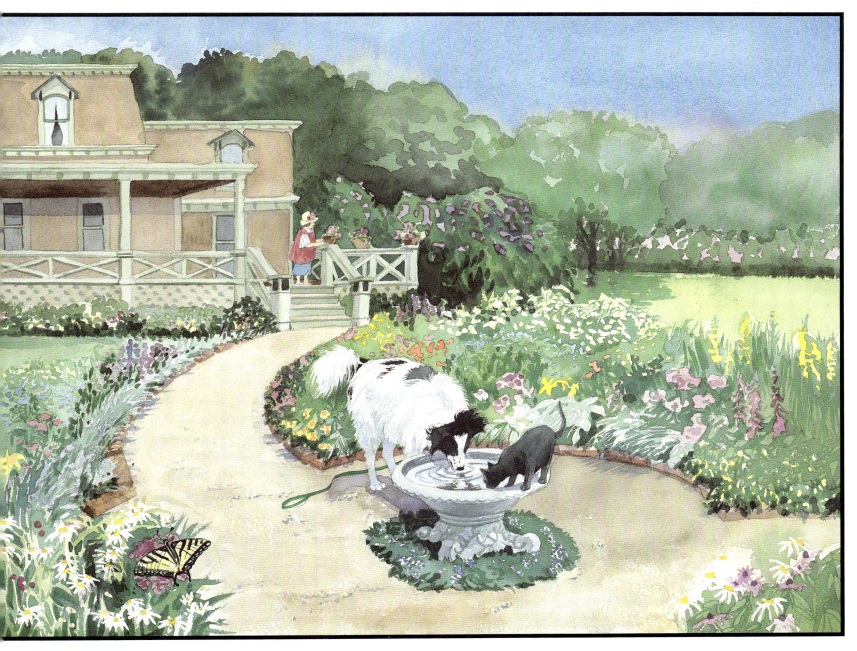

The sun came out, and Nathaniel watched a butterfly flutter towards the house. Oh, no! Old Mrs. Crowell was at the door! Nathaniel was too scared to run. But the old woman smiled and said, "I recognize Jeff, so you must be Nathaniel."

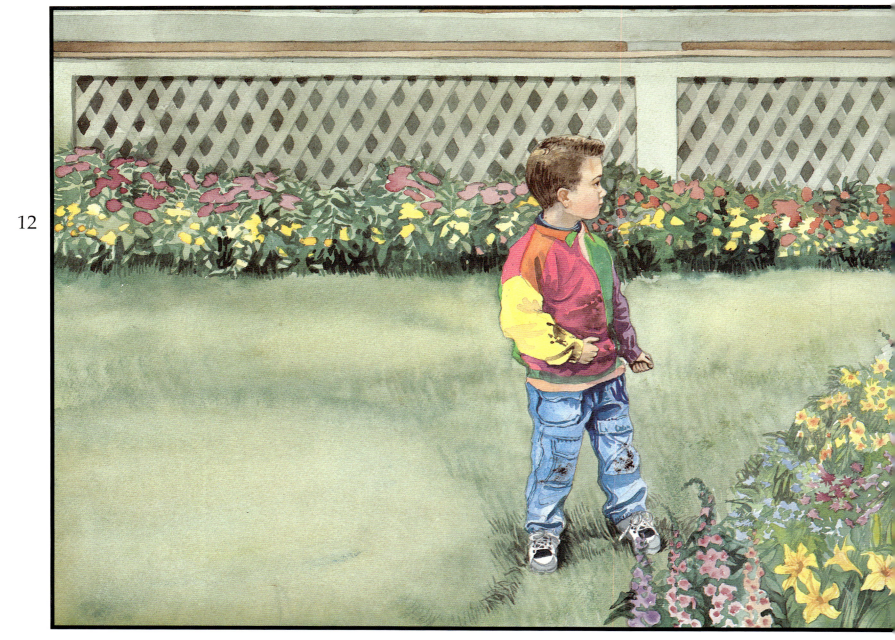

12

"You know my name?" asked Nathaniel. He thought old Mrs. Crowell looked nice in her sun hat, gardening apron, and blue skirt. She didn't seem scary at all, but he still wasn't sure.

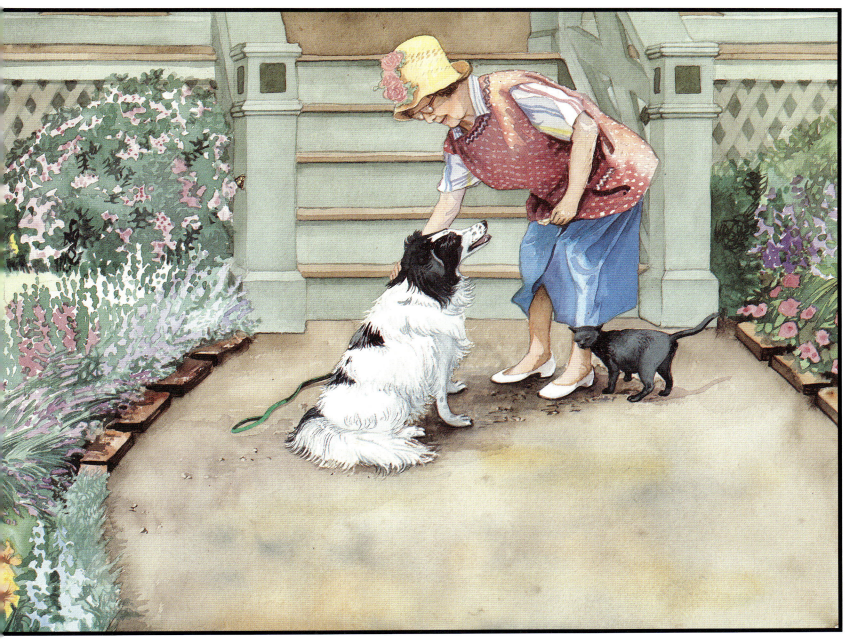

"Your mother has been here to buy some wreaths, and she told me all about you," said Mrs. Crowell. She called Jeff and Shadow up to the porch for some cheese. Jeff wagged his tail and even licked old Mrs. Crowell's face. Nathaniel thought, "She doesn't seem mean, she seems friendly."

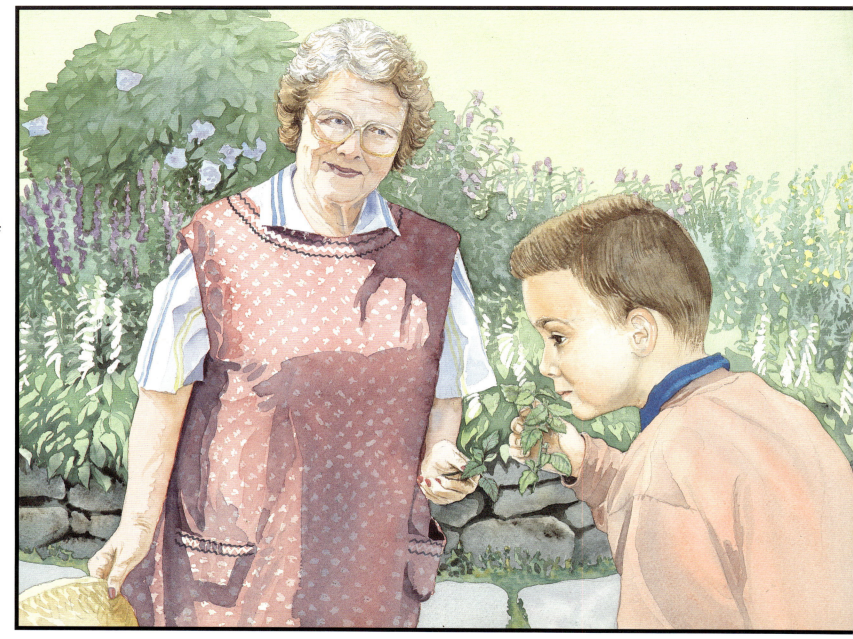

"Come, I'll show you my gardens," said Mrs. Crowell. "But, first, why don't you hang your jacket on the line to dry." Nathaniel's jacket was torn and muddy from his fall. As they walked, Mrs. Crowell picked leaves from some of her plants and asked Nathaniel to smell them. They smelled just like their names. There was lemon balm, orange mint, and rose geranium.

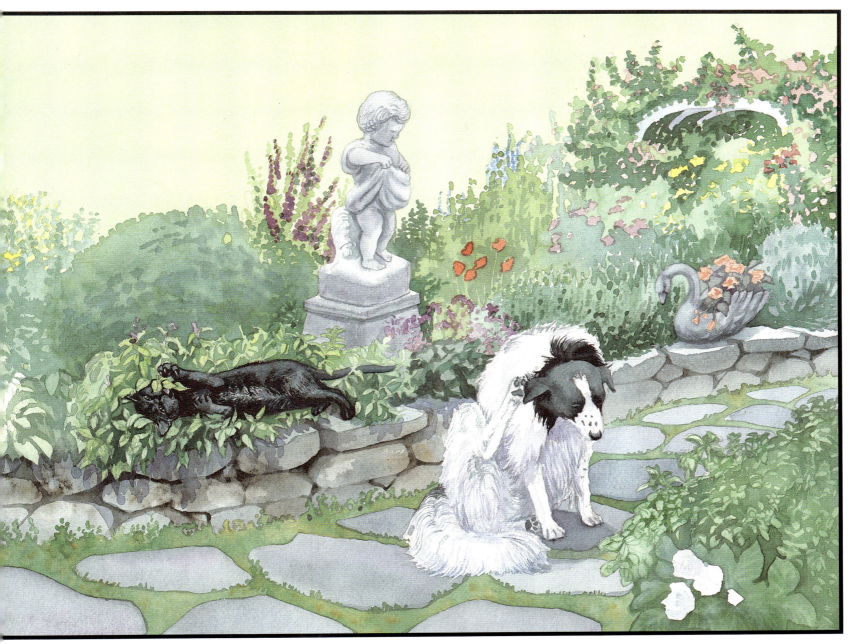

Some plants looked like their names. There was silver mound, lavender, golden thyme, blue sage, and pink yarrow. There was a plant for Shadow called catnip, and one for Jeff called pennyroyal. Mrs. Crowell said pennyroyal could help get rid of fleas. Nathaniel thought, "Mrs. Crowell knows all sorts of good things."

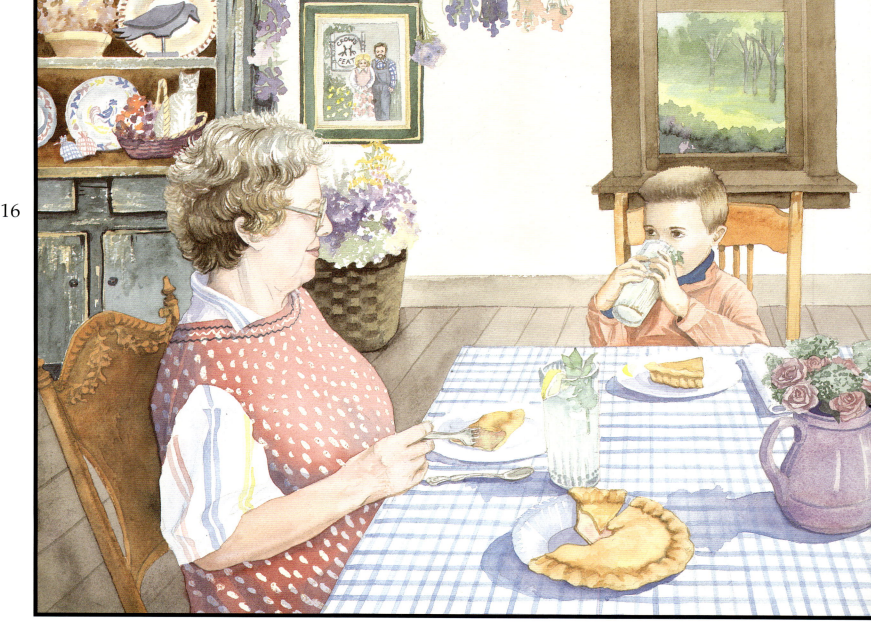

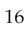ome with me. I'll make you some special tea to go with my famous rhubarb pie," said Mrs. Crowell. She made a mint tulip with mint leaves, lemon balm, and lemonade. Then she cut a big piece of rhubarb pie for each of them.

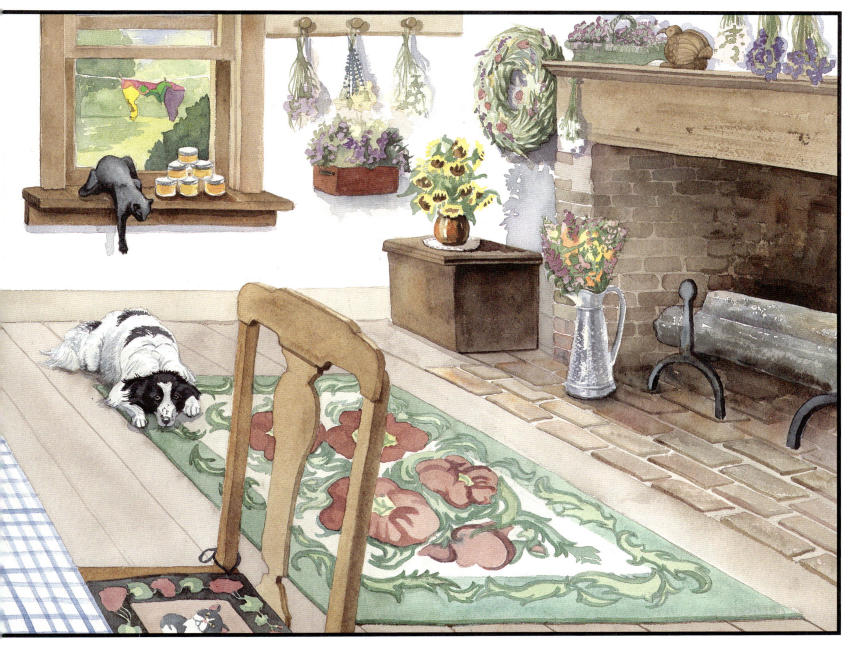

"Do you live alone here?" Nathaniel asked. "Yes," she replied. "Now I do. My husband and I—I call him Cro—ran the farm for fifty years. The farm's name is Crow's Feat. Cro lives in a nursing home now, and all our children are married and have moved away."

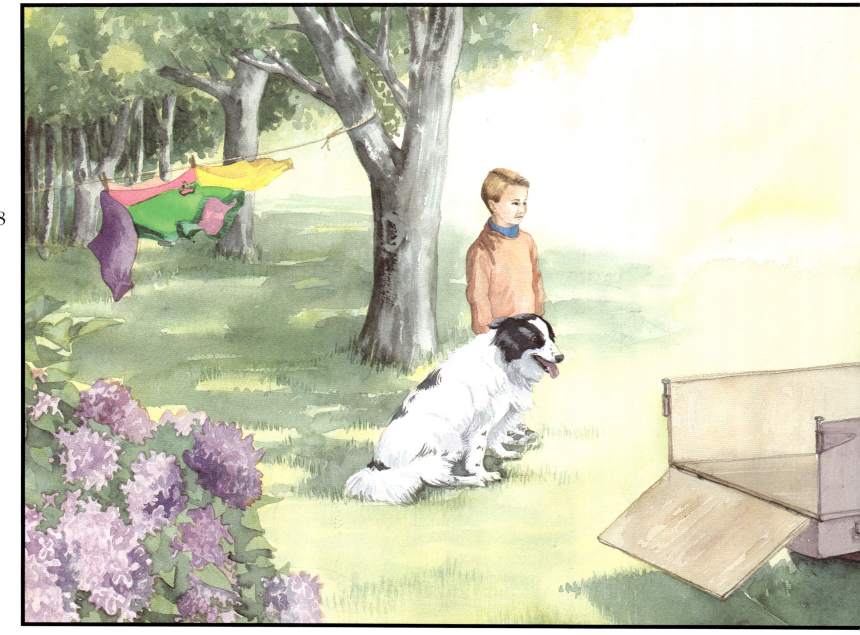

18

"Now, let's go pick some flowers for Cro and his friends at the nursing home. You three hop in, and I'll give you a ride to the cutting garden."

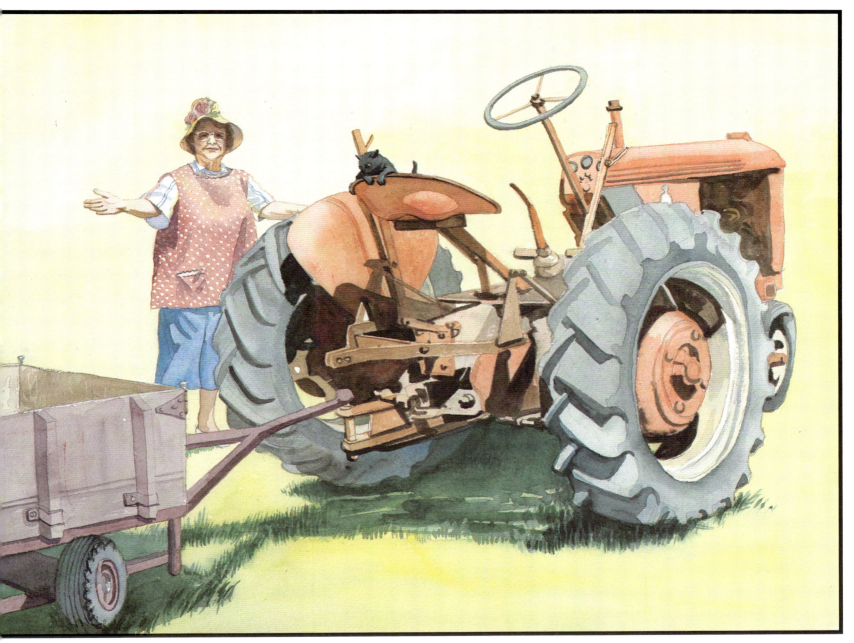

To Nathaniel's surprise, Mrs. Crowell pointed to a tractor and waved them all into the trailer. Then she climbed up, turned the key, and started to drive.

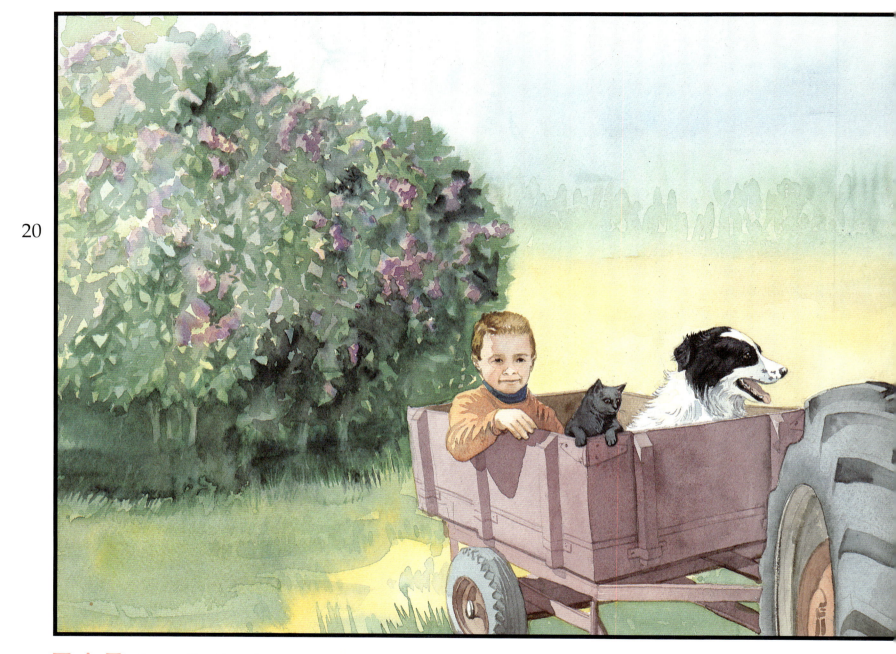

While Jeff, Shadow, and Nathaniel rode behind Mrs. Crowell, Nathaniel wondered why he had been afraid of her.

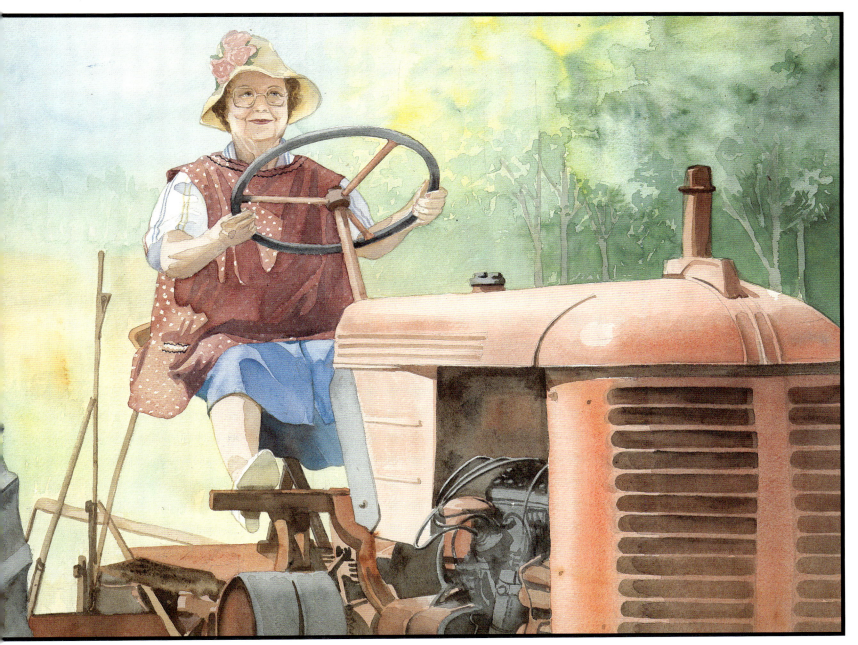

She had some wrinkles and her fingers were kind of knobby, but she had bright blue eyes, and she smiled a lot. He liked her.

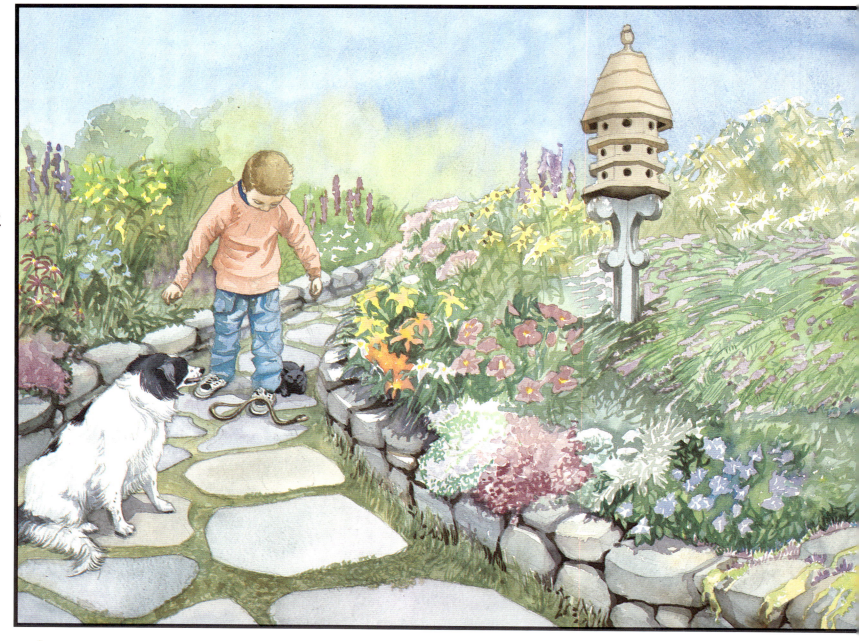

s Nathaniel was about to pick a yellow lily, a snake slithered over his sneaker and scared the breath right out of him. Mrs. Crowell gently caught the snake and showed Nathaniel how to handle it. "Most snakes are harmless. They won't hurt you. They eat insects, and that's good for my garden," she explained.

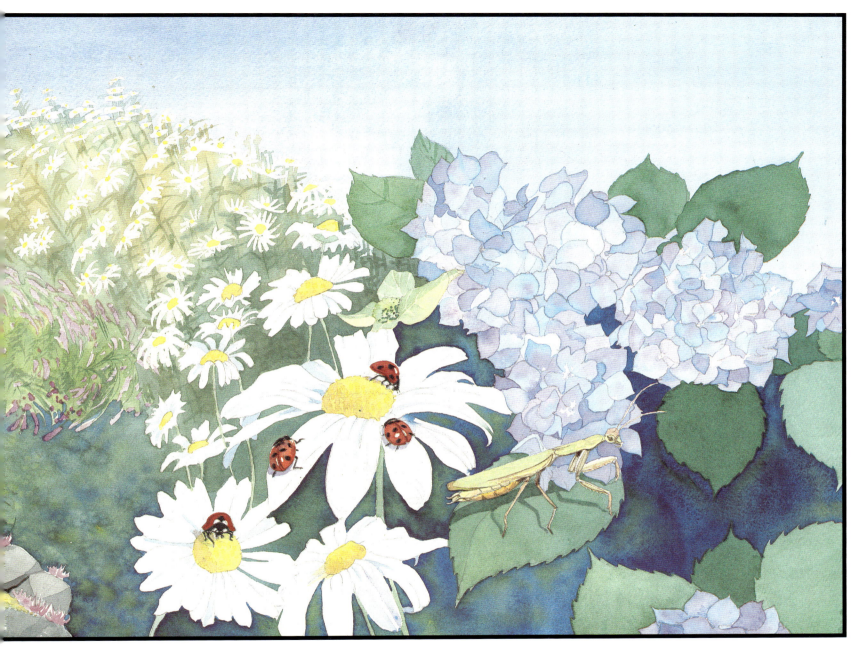

She showed Nathaniel a ladybug and a praying mantis. "Ladybugs are a symbol of good luck," she said. "They eat aphids and mites and other insects that harm plants. The praying mantis lives on caterpillars, flies, and some kinds of moths."

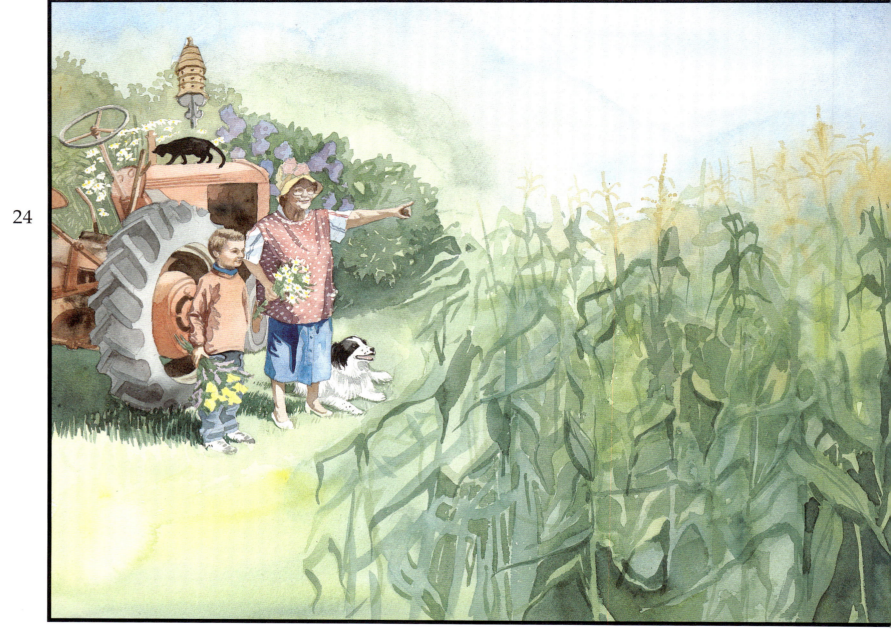

"How do you know so much?" asked Nathaniel. "I've worked in gardens and with flowers all my life, and that's a long time because I'm an old lady. I love to learn new things every day," answered Mrs. Crowell.

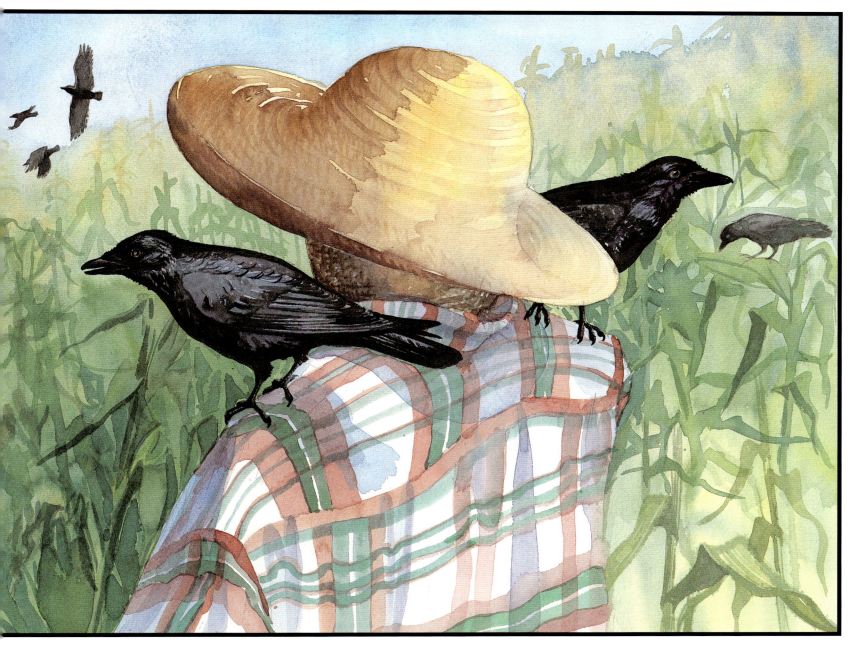

In the cornfield Nathaniel saw a hay-stuffed hat and shirt on a pole. Big black birds stood on each shoulder. They reminded Nathaniel of the shadows in his bedroom. Mrs. Crowell sighed. "A scarecrow doesn't hurt the crows, but it *is* supposed to frighten them. My scarecrow isn't even frightening. I have to think of something to scare the crows away or they'll ruin my corn."

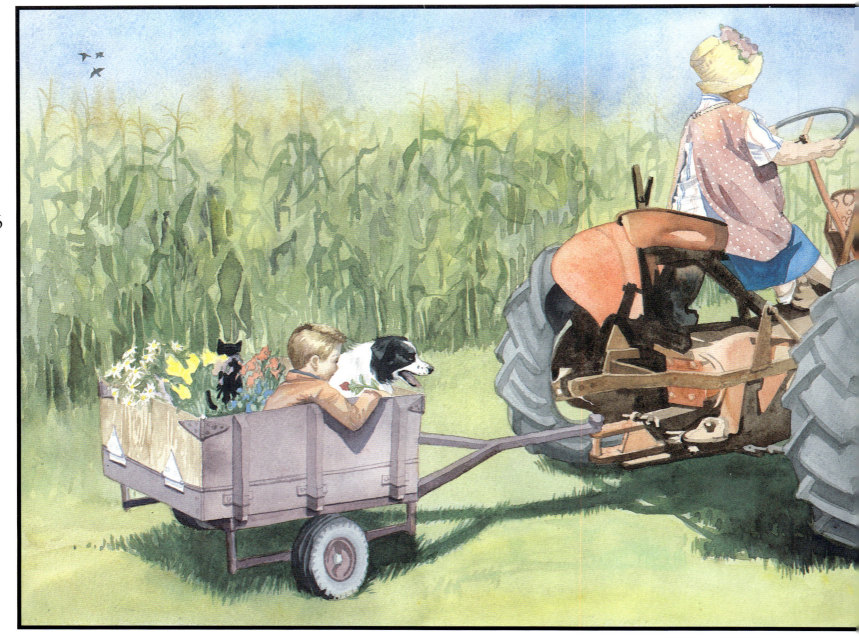

athaniel wished he could think of a way to help Mrs. Crowell. She had been so nice to him. On their way back to the house, he saw his jacket dancing wildly on the clothesline. As it filled up with air, the sleeves bent and straightened just like arms.

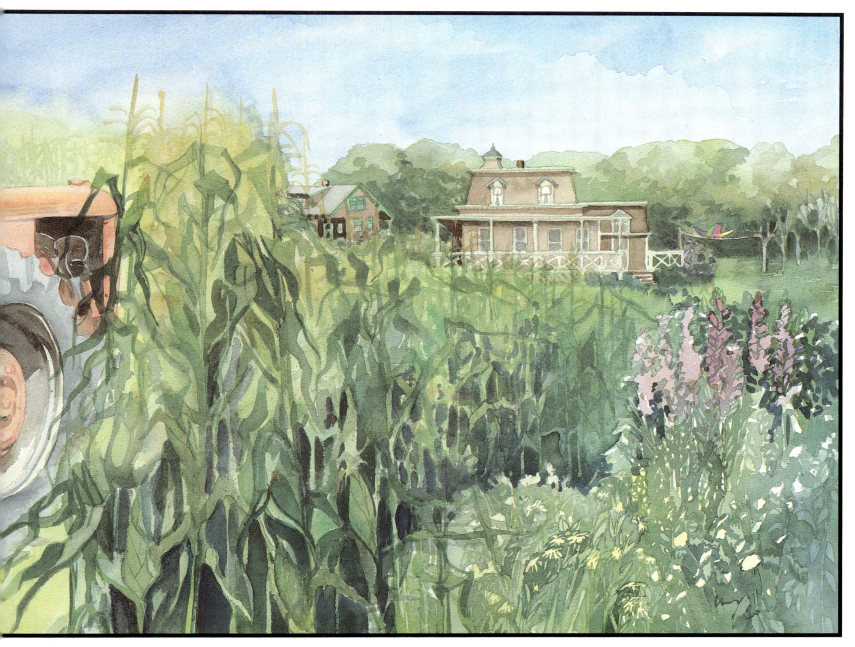

"How about my jacket? My mother wants to throw it away anyhow. In school we made windsocks. Let's make one for the cornfield! My jacket's torn and muddy, but it would be perfect. I'll show you how," insisted Nathaniel. "We need a hanger, string, and sewing things."

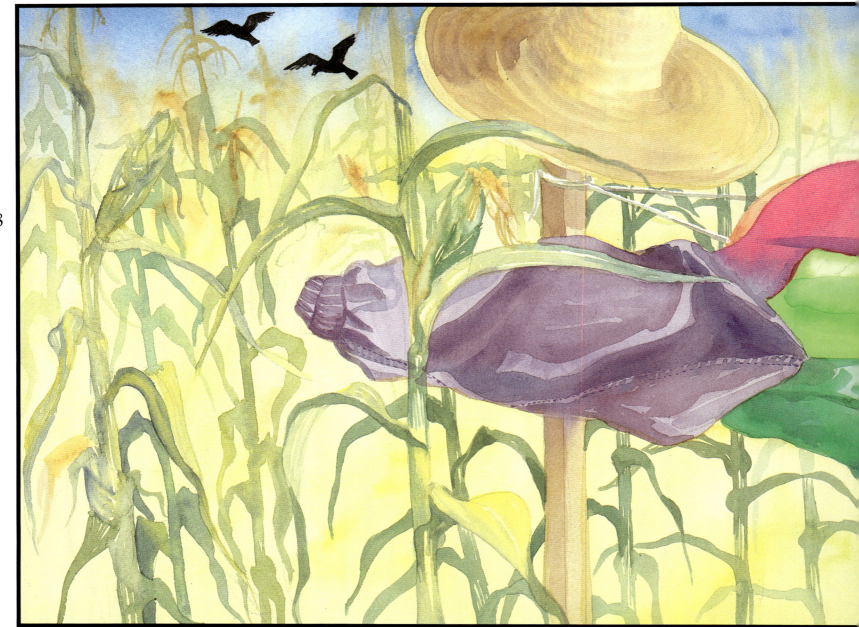

athaniel shaped the coat hanger into a circle, and Mrs. Crowell sewed the jacket around it. They sewed the sleeves closed and made the waist smaller. Then they tied it to the scarecrow pole with string. The jacket filled up with air and moved with the wind.

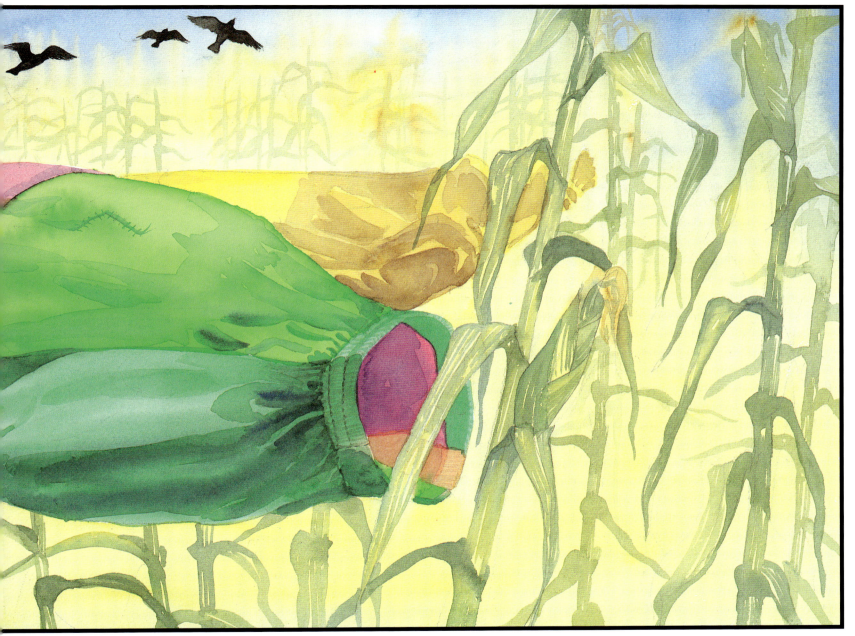

The jacket moved so fast and was so bright and noisy when it crinkled that all the crows were frightened and flew off to find other food. "What a great idea, Nathaniel! You shall have the first ear of corn when it's ripe!" exclaimed Mrs. Crowell. "I'm so glad we met." "I'm glad, too," answered Nathaniel.

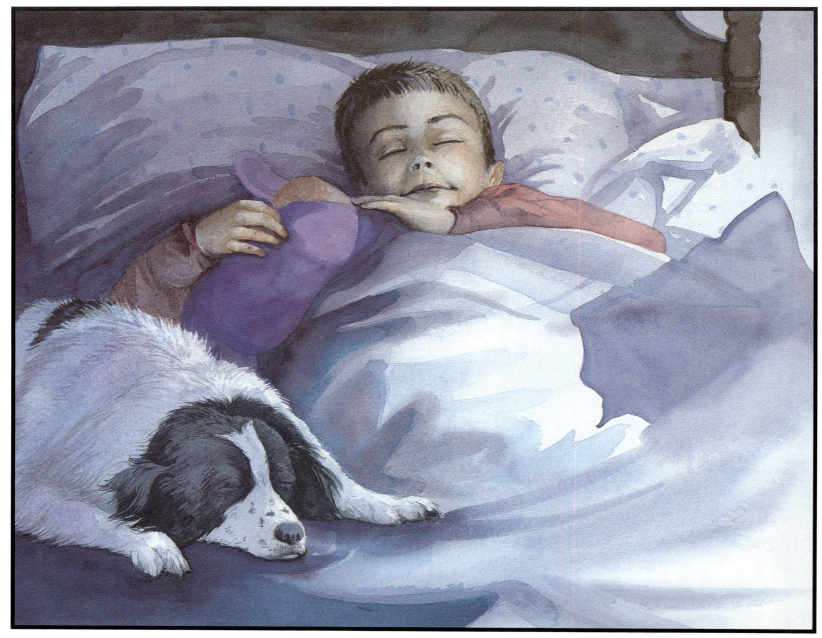

When Nathaniel got home, his mother asked him where his jacket was. He explained that he had given it to a friend who needed it. In bed that night, when the shadows moved and the scary crow began to appear, Nathaniel wasn't frightened. He knew the shadow came from his new friend's house. Pretty soon, he and Mrs. Crowell would enjoy the first corn of the harvest.

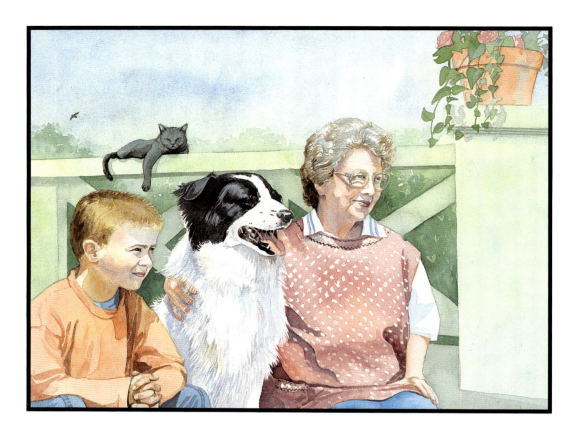

My paintings were done in watercolor from three very accommodating models, my mother, Elizabeth MacDonald, my nephew, Seamus MacDonald, and Jeff the Dog.

My thanks to the following Westport, Massachusetts, residents for their contributions:

Mr. and Mrs. Ben Gifford—Nathaniel's house
Mr. and Mrs. Ralph Guild—Mrs. Crowell's house
Al Lees—pie and lemonade
Russell Hart—tractor
Jack Pacheco—trailer
Paul Costa—corn
Bill Connelly—jacket
Courtyards in Tiverton, Rhode Island—garden objects
Local crows

Betsy Douglas MacDonald